SEDATION DENTISTRY: THE ULTIMATE PATIENT GUIDE

*Your Complete How-To Guide to Understanding
and Overcoming Your Fear of the Dentist,
Anesthesia, Drills, Needles and Dental Tools
Once and for All With or Without Sedation.*

Rene Piedra

Disclaimer

The statements in this book have not been evaluated by the Food and Drug Administration. This book is not intended in any way to provide medical advice or to be a substitute for medical advice. The information here does not represent medical advice. If you're seeking medical advice, contact a medical or dental practitioner. All content provided is for informational purposes only and represents an expression of opinions by the author. Products, services, and information in this book are not intended to diagnose, treat, cure, or prevent any disease. If you have a severe medical condition, see a physician or dentist of your choice.

While every effort has been made to ensure the information provided is accurate, the author, publisher, and distributer make no warranties with respect to the accuracy or completeness of the contents of the book, nor assume any responsibility for errors or omissions.

In no event will be author and/or marketer be liable for any direct, indirect, incidental, consequential or other loss or damage arising out of the use of this book by any person, regardless of whether or not they were informed of the possibility of damages in advance.

ISBN: 0692453415
ISBN 13: 9780692453414
Library of Congress Control Number: 2015908478
New Era Dentistry, Miami, FL

Dear Dr. Piedra,

    I want to take a moment to apologize for canceling on you again. I have driven to your office four times and have not been able to get out of the car because I am simply terrified of dentists.

    Again, I apologize for canceling our appointment again. Let me tell you a bit about my situation. When I was seven my mother took me to the dentist outside of the town where we lived to pull a tooth. When he started, I told the dentist I was feeling pain. He told my mother that it was not true, that I was just being a baby, that it was normal to feel what I was feeling. I felt every tug and pull, and to make matters worse he broke the tooth while he was pulling it. I don't want to recall what I saw, but ever since then I have been really afraid of going to the dentist. It's affecting my marriage in many ways but I won't get into it. My husband made the first appointment for me with your office and I honestly tried to go. I have an abscess that has come back. My husband tells me I look angry all the time and I never smile.

    I can say that I haven't smiled almost ever. I hope you don't think I'm a nut case. I am very embarrassed about my teeth, about not going to the dentist, and I know it's affecting me in many ways, but I simply can't do it.

    I called my doctor and he's given me antibiotics. I have an appointment for next month and

I am having my husband take the day off so he can come in with me. I am your nightmare client but this time I'm coming in. I hope you can help.

Once again, my apologies.

Sincerely,

Marsha B.

This book is dedicated to the countless Marshas who are afraid of the dentist to one degree or another, who long for healthy teeth and gums for a lifetime. To their transformation.

CONTENTS

INTRODUCTION

"I learned that courage was not the absence of
fear, but the triumph over it. The brave man
is not he who does not feel afraid, but he who
conquers that fear."

— NELSON MANDELA

Hi, my name is Dr. Rene Piedra, and I have spent the better part of the last seventeen years of my professional career treating a broad spectrum of fearful dental patients – from the mildly apprehensive to the most terrified of patients – gaining national attention and earning accolades in the field of fearful dental patient care.

Having treated over 35,000 patients, I've created various systems for allaying those fears to the end of bringing lifelong sound oral health to this underserved and needy population while introducing revolutionary pain- and fear-dispelling instrumentation and procedures for them. In the field of treating the fearful patient, my systems have involved approaches from bringing around even the mildly apprehensive dentophobe by way of specialized bedside manner systems to successfully treating even more at-risk special needs patients.

My goal – and the goal of this book – is to enable you, no matter your degree of apprehension or fear of the dentist, needles, pain, or even embarrassment, to bring you the tools you need to maintain much-needed oral health for sound well-being. If you have ever avoided going to the dentist, or if you continue to stay away from the dentist for any reason, then this book was written just for you.

That's why we're here today, so let's get started!

1

WHAT IS FEAR OF THE DENTIST?

"The disease is painless; it's the cure that hurts"

— KATHERINE WHITEHORN

What is Fear?

Fear is perhaps the most primitive animal emotion that is inherent in all of us. It is an unpleasant emotion sparked by the belief that a particular person or a particular situation is dangerous or likely to cause pain. The mind perceives someone or something as a threat that must be avoided. A stimulant perceived by the mind by any of the five senses sets off a chain reaction within the body, more commonly known as a "flight or fight response," and the entire body along with the mind engages into avoidance mode. Blood from the digestive system is instantly redirected to necessary parts of the body; the heart starts to beat fast, rushing oxygenated blood to the brain and muscles in order for the individual to escape the threat and survive. Like mating, you can see this in all animals, all geared toward furthering the survival of the individual and the species. Though it must be said that as far as animal instincts go, "fear" isn't nearly as fun.

We are all afraid of something to one degree or another. Taking a test, approaching a person whom we find attractive, and speaking in public are all extremely common sources of fear, but there are ways to keep fear at bay, and there are even methods to eradicate fear entirely. Although as a species we have developed logic and intellect sufficient enough to keep most of our emotions under control (including this most primitive of emotions), events from our past, both experienced and learned from others, impinge on how we think and react. To a great degree this survival emotion can indeed jeopardize our survival instead of helping us, especially when not controlled. It goes beyond just being scared of the dark or not getting on a roller coaster for fear of heights; fear can take on less obvious manifestations like prejudice and racism. Again, these can be learned or they can be a consequence of past experiences recorded and embedded subconsciously the mind.

One of the most interesting characteristics of fear is that conscientious, logical and accurate thinking and perception go out the window and fear takes control of the individual's response, actions, thinking and conclusions one way or another. The fearful individual is not thinking clearly, and is making decisions that are actually counterproductive toward his continued well-being. I'm personally of the opinion that the balance has to shift away from fear by way of self-control for a sentient species like ours to further develop its intellectual and logical abilities toward a more advanced, currently nonexistent ability, emotion or sense.

But alas this is not a treatise on human intellect and its advancement. Fear is a response which controls the individual, causing one to react to a particular situation or stimulant based on a similar previous stimulation from which one unwittingly "learned" to protect himself. Fear is a mental and bodily emotion that we continue to use in this moment of evolution as a protective mechanism to propagate our life and existence. Without self-control, this emotion will control us to the end of hurting us by way of inaccurate and sub-optimal decisions and actions.

Media, Painful Experiences and Parents

Not many people think of the dentist as the kindly benefactor portrayed by Norman Rockwell. In fact, going purely by depictions of dentists in the media – from the scary movie "The Dentist" to Steve Martin's psychotic turn in "Little Shop of Horrors" – it's amazing that anyone *ever* goes to the dentist!

Fear can be a result of past painful experiences, it can be taught to us intentionally or passed on inadvertently, or we may more commonly put ourselves in the path of communication that instills fear in us. Many of us are completely unaware about why we are fearful of certain things. If you took a two-year-old and an adult and pinched them for the first time in their lives, let's say for illustrative purposes with a paper clip, the discomfort experienced by the two-year-old would be exponentially more than that felt by the adult. From that point forward, perhaps for the rest of his life, the pinched two-year-old would react in avoidance of whatever reminded him of a pinch or paper-clip, the aversion stimulus, as he would have at the age of two. Meanwhile, the adult who was pinched for the first time as an adult would not make much of the visual, tactical or audio reminder of the pinch. Many times we react illogically and "without reason" to someone or something and it is simply a sense – sight, smell, sound or touch – causing whatever experience is embedded in the subconscious to fire up into protection mode unconsciously. Here again we have inexplicable fights, jealousy, psychosomatic pain, etc.

Parents can also influence our perception of the world around us and make us fearful through their own fear. I can tell you I was never afraid of heights until my mother forbid me to go near a railing on a fifth floor balcony. More of my own fear of heights and some comic relief later, but I have witnessed parents tell their children, "If you don't behave, I'm going to take you to the doctor to get an injection." Seriously?!

I really get a kick out of being asked by a patient I've seen the movie "The Dentist." Don't get me wrong, I really enjoy horror flicks myself, but even I get the willies when they depict particular situations within the movie involving blood, pain, and drills. Why do we purposefully put ourselves in a situation where we can get scared?

Another situation we put ourselves in which terrorizes us is watching the news. When I was growing up we only had ten channels to choose from, with only three news channels, each airing just four hours of news daily at most. With so many channels competing for ratings which are necessary for them to price their commercial time, the scope of informational media has shifted from journalism to entertainment. Now, in my neck of the woods there's only so much you can say, for example, about a hurricane. The information that I need is for the hurricane is: when will it be here, how strong are the winds and how long will it linger if it does hit? I can be told this information at most in a matter of three minutes. But how they manage to broadcast 48 hours of nonstop hurricane coverage boggles my mind. The same information chewed up and regurgitated in countless ways. This is the modus operandi of modern day media: the use of rousing or shocking language and stories with the intent of provoking public interest and excitement in a congested business heavily competing for public attention (at the expense of accuracy, I may add) is the news of the day, pun intended.

If the information is not consciously scrutinized by the viewer, and we rarely do, the net result is fear. I really believe that the thought fabric of our society is media driven by way of fear, which again, leads to inaccurate reasoning, decisions, actions and attitudes.

How does this connect to dentophobia? How's this for a surprising fact: I have patients sleeping through root canals. In fact, the norm is that patients actually doze off during root canals, but when was the last time you heard that a root canal was painless or that the procedure was pleasant? All you hear is that root canals are painful, and even men tell me they would rather go through childbirth than get a root canal. I usually respond that they'll need to consult an entirely different sort of medical professional for that particular procedure.

Perception and Fear- Dentistry vs. Mixed Martial Arts Cage Fighting

Let me start off by saying that for some, jumping into a small cage with a seven-foot, hulking martial arts professional fighter and duking it out for twelve minutes is not as scary as going to the dentist. I always tell the story about a patient whom I encountered in 2001 who made a living from fixing slot machines around the country and around the world. His passion, though, was cage fighting. This guy was nearly seven feet tall, I kid you not, with a shoulder width possibly twice mine to the point where I actually had to adjust how I sat when I laid him back to examine him. If he wasn't on steroids he was doubling up on his Wheaties and spinach, a gargantuan Johnny Weissmuller-type who could eat Hulk Hogan for breakfast.. Now, I'm not a small guy and not much intimidates me, but let's just say that I had every intention of making the dental exam experience for this self-described fearful patient as quick and easy as possible for his benefit and mine.

I have a habit of placing my hand on the patient's shoulder or arm when I'm speaking with them and prior to going into their mouth, and when I did that with this patient he continued to talk and converse. Normally the high-fear patient has certain idiosyncrasies that indicate their mood and attitude, but this gentleman seemed un-bothered at this point. So, I laid him back, asked him to open his mouth, and the moment I touched his gum with my gloved finger, his entire body elevated nearly two feet off the chair, all horizontally and at once. I can say that I have never flown backward in startle like I did that day. My assistant nearly collapsed.

The fact is that what I had done, which was place my finger on his gum before anything, caused him to think that it was already hurting. He told me it hurt. I looked again, thinking that perhaps there was something patho-logic going on in the area I palpated, but it was indeed normal. He responded in kind to everything I touched. He was predisposed by fear to such a degree that he per-ceived that what I was doing was painful.

This guy was used to getting hit, punched, kicked and choked all the time without reservation, but had such a perception of oral pain that he reacted with an inaccurate emotional and physical response which had nothing to do with physical pain and everything to do with fear. Not that

I don't occasionally use the line that I subdued a pro cage fighter with nothing but my little finger.

Wile E. Coyote's Safe Landing

Wile E. Coyote, Elvis Presley, Muhammad Ali, Ronald Reagan and I all share a common fear. Back in 2000 I took up my childhood dream of flying. If you're not familiar with the process of getting a private pilot's license, after learning the theory of flying and after your instructor is confident that you can take off and land properly, then you do what's called a cross-country flight, meaning flying from one airport to another airport. So I was all ready to do my first cross-country flight, and after plotting and charting the course and having it okayed by my instructor, I got in the aircraft and I took off. I turned away from the airport and headed from Miami to Naples. The problem began as soon as I started over the Everglades when I suddenly remembered that I was afraid of heights.

Boy, did that become a problem! Although I was confident being alone in the aircraft, the sudden realization that I was all by myself over an area where I couldn't land sent me into a panic. Then I made the mistake of looking out the window to my side and looked at the ground. Just like in the cartoons, I felt like Wile E. Coyote about to plummet to my doom, and literally saw the Everglades move at me and away from me for the longest ten seconds of my life. It was sheer terror and I literally feared for my life. What a bad feeling it was to feel completely helpless, alone and trapped while aware that nothing bad was actually occurring and that I was in no way in control of myself nor my feelings. I suddenly remembered from when I was fifteen and taking my scuba lessons that most tragedies occur when one loses focus and panics in the midst of an emergency. I forced myself to bring my attention to the present moment at hand – as opposed to staying in the moment from the past that had been re-stimulated – and I soon gained control of myself. Although I had not lost control of the aircraft, the overwhelming fear that took my attention to something other than control of myself and the aircraft could have resulted in tragedy.

We are all afraid of something and it boggles my mind when I hear a patient complain about a previous dentist telling them to not be a baby. I know what it is to be afraid. To have a dentist invalidate a patient and say, "Oh, no need to be afraid, it's not going to hurt" simply falls of deaf ears as it is not real. I understand fear. What is real to you is what is real. If I were to point out a pen and told you that it was actually a paperclip, it just would not compute. It is not real to you. To have a dentist tell you "Oh don't worry, this is not going to hurt" is simply not real and you will be just as afraid, possibly even more afraid knowing that the person about to anesthetize you actually DOES NOT understand. I laugh when a healthcare professional tells a patient who will have an instrument used on them not to worry, that it won't hurt. Perhaps that is completely real to an operator who in a rote way is performing the same procedure all day long, but that's cold comfort to the patient.

You and I are not alone. Some well-liked and admired personalities in history have grappled with their own fears. Bela Lugosi, the much feared "Dracula," was afraid of blood. Basketball legend Michael Jordan was afraid of water. Giants of state Julius Caesar, Napoléon Bonaparte, and Alexander the Great, were reported to suffer from *ailurophobia*, fear of cats. Frederick Chopin, one of my favorite composers, was afraid of being buried alive, while Walt Disney was afraid of mice.

People who avoid the dentist can be afraid of dental treatment, pain, needles, not being able to get numb, the sound of the drill, what they've heard about root canals, embarrassment, blood, losing teeth, drowning, not being able to breathe, bad news, tight quarters, not being able to get up and go as they please or being confined, germs, shaming lectures, or laying back while a complete stranger uses metal tools on their head...to name a few.

Whatever the cause or exact nature of your fear, this book is your ticket to move you from fear to beautiful, healthy teeth and gums for a lifetime.

2

WHAT DOES DENTISTRY HAVE TO DO WITH MY LIFE AND LIFESTYLE?

"There is no such thing as bravery; only degrees of fear."

— JOHN WAINWRIGHT

I graduated from dental school in 1998, and at the time I heard to my surprise that dental disease led to heart attacks. I thought of it as a bit of malarkey and somewhat of an unfounded sales pitch at the time, but as I continued my studies I came to learn that the correlations between sound oral health and general health preceded through an understanding of the opposite effect, the oral manifestations of general health and disease. Indeed, there are general health issues that affect the mouth and visa versa. There are less obvious concerns involved with poor oral health, from psychological to social which can lead to sub-optimal health and lifestyle.

What Does Diabetes Have to Do With My Teeth?

A basic understanding of diabetes is necessary to understand its role in keeping your teeth as well as the role that poor oral health has on developing diabetes. Diabetes Mellitus (DM) is a group of disorders that share certain characteristics, including impaired metabolism of fat and carbohydrates or an altered tolerance for glucose. In diabetes, there is an elevation in the amount of glucose in the blood which if controlled or uncontrolled may detrimentally affect other parts of the body.

The problem with controlling blood glucose levels is that the body's normal capability to repair itself is impaired. We've all heard how someone with DM may have had a sore that took much longer to heal than normal, or that someone lost their sight or even a limb as a result of an inability to control blood glucose levels and impaired wound healing.

This presents an important problem within the mouth. The structures which keep the teeth in place and attached to the jaw bone are affected with diabetes. What happens is that the body can start to lose bone around the teeth, a disease called periodontitis or gum disease. There is a loss of the bone that makes up the structure that hold the teeth in place. Worse yet, this is a disease that is not felt and once started cannot be cured. The person unaware of what's happening ends up losing bone little by little, and the net result is loose teeth that need to be removed. There is a 59% greater incidence of severe periodontal disease in diabetics than in the general population, and diabetics suffer from greater rates of tooth loss as well. If fact, periodontal disease is the leading cause of tooth loss in the United States.

The flip side is that increased glucose levels cause certain inflammatory proteins to be released into the blood. These inflammatory proteins cause a cascade of events that can in turn lead to insulin intolerance and diabetes.

So what does all this mean? It means that if you are diabetic it is critical that you frequent the dentist as you are at a higher risk of developing periodontal disease and lose your teeth, and if you have poor oral health – you don't floss nightly or don't frequent the dentist along with or in the absence of some other factors – it can lead to diabetes. It is important to note that 75% of Americans have some level of periodontal disease. I understand this information can be alarming but my purpose here is prevention of health problems.

In short, you need to go to the dentist to get the sticky, invisible, bacteria-laden plaque on the teeth removed to avoid a slew of possible conditions.

What's the Deal With Not Going to the Dentist and Having a Stroke or Heart Attack?

In the United States, twelve Million heart attacks occur each year, resulting in nearly 30% of all deaths. Studies indicate that people suffering from severe gum disease are twice as likely to suffer from cardiovascular disease; that is, stroke, heart attack, atherosclerosis, arrhythmia and heart failure. The predominant thought is that bacteria that live under the gums as a result of poor hygiene, meaning a lack of personal and professional care can become blood borne and colonize fatty plaque residues that occur on the inner walls of a blood vessels, causing these plaque residues to disengage from the inner wall of the blood vessel. The plaque then travels throughout the blood stream until it reaches a blood vessel with smaller diameter than itself, thereby sealing up the vessel from that point on and leaving the tissue of the heart, brain or other organ deprived of oxygen. This is where the mobility occurs. Although exact causes like bacteria types involved and the exact sequence of events are not well established, for the last 40 years periodontitis has increasingly been regarded as a risk factor for cardiovascular disease.

While I am not suggesting that if someone doesn't floss or frequent the dentist they will suffer a heart attack, I am underscoring the fact that good gum and periodontal health is becoming an accepted key goal that can contribute to reducing strokes, heart attacks, atherosclerosis and the like.

Other systemic conditions have been attributed to periodontal disease such as low birthweight babies, respiratory disease, osteoporosis and even cancer. In fact research has concluded that while men without periodontal disease are still at risk of cancer, all things being equal, there is a 49% increase in the probability of developing kidney cancer, a 54% increase in the chances of developing pancreatic cancer, and a 30% increase in developing blood associated cancers.

Okay, I know this is a lot of scary stuff. But that's a good thing to keep in mind! While I don't want to keep you up at nights worrying about your oral health, it's important to remember that the real fear lies in *not* going to the dentist.

Is Not Going to The Dentist Keeping Me Fat?

Well, it can. In my book, *The Ultimate Snoring and Apnea Solution: The Simple Solution for Easily Adding Years to Your Life and Marriage Through Snoring Cessation,* I touch on the factors related to snoring and obstructive sleep apnea, a condition the general public is generally unaware of, and how addressing it can have a remarkable effect on your lifestyle. So while thinking about going to the dentist might be keeping you up at night, it turns out that not taking care of your oral health can have an even worse impact on your sleep! Let's briefly examine how sleep apnea relates to visiting the dentist.

What happens when you sleep is that the muscles that keep your airway open relax, causing the oxygen level in your blood to decrease while carbon dioxide levels increase. This has an effect on your cardiovascular system and your GI system, and had many other implications too numerous to mention here. One important repercussion of snoring and sleep apnea is its effect on the endocrine system.

In the body of a sufferer of sleep apnea, cortisol levels build up, leading to increased stress, while at the same time growth hormone and thyroid stimulating hormones decrease. In addition, testosterone levels in women increase, but there are two particular hormones that will answer the question in this subchapter.

There is a hormone called leptin produced by fat cells that signals the brain that you are full. What happens with obstructive sleep apnea (OSA) and associated snoring is that a leptin resistance occurs where this signal is impeded and the person tends to eat until engorged. This of course leads to many other problems described in the book, but increased weight is one of them.

Another hormone that is affected is ghrelin, also known as the "hunger hormone." It acts on the same part of the brain as leptin and is released when the stomach is empty and its secretion stops when the stomach muscle is stretched, telling the brain that we are full. Have you ever heard of waiting fifteen minutes before eating more to give the body time to feel full? The problem presented in patients with OSA is that there is an elevation in the secretion of ghrelin, signaling the brain that one is still hungry. By the way, the effect of OSA on the thyroid also contributes to weight gain.

Interrupted sleep has more direct detrimental effects on one's health, too. Hitting the snooze button five times in the morning and waking up tired because you haven't had a restful sleep does not help much with motivation in getting the necessary exercise for dropping weight. Here too, OSA affects one's weight.

So what the heck does any of this have to do with the dentist? The American Academy of Sleep Medicine stated in the January 2006 issue of the journal *Sleep* that oral appliances are the first treatment option for patients with mild to moderate sleep apnea. An oral appliance is a small, relatively comfortable device that a person sleeps with that easily allows their airway to remain open when the muscles around their necks and mouth relax while they sleep. The right apnea appliance can eliminate or significantly reduce snoring and apnea in cases where it is indicated. A medical physician cannot make these for you, only a qualified dentist with advanced education in the field can and should treat this.

How Is Poor Oral Health Affecting Me Socially?

Avoiding the dentist can affect you in a number of ways, only some of which you may be aware of. For example, a person working with public can be embarrassed about the way their teeth look or their breath smells. This may be manifested in an inability to smile because of differences in symmetry and color in their smile. Moreover, comfort level in social settings such as meeting people, working with people, applying for a job, socializing with people, or approaching in a romantic scenario may be very uncomfortable and some may even avoid those situations because of their embarrassment over the condition of their teeth. Introversion – that is, having your attention focused on yourself – can kill success when dealing with others.

The vast majority of people who avoid the dentist are painfully aware of these shortcomings; however, some are completely unaware. I have indeed met people were not aware of the differences in color of their teeth that gave them an asymmetric smile. Although I'm used to it and it doesn't bother me whatsoever, halitosis or bad breath can be obnoxious to others, and being unaware of this in social and in work settings can have a detrimental effect on everything from meeting people to making a sale.

Luckily in today's dentistry all of these conditions can be easily addressed in a non-painful, non-stimulative dental setting. Before the end of this book you will have the know-how to put any of these adverse effects behind you.

This leads me to the importance of a smile. I hate to address it like that because it seems like common sense, but it definitely warrants a few words. Consider the last time you came across someone who just did not smile. What impression did that person make on you? Perhaps they were angry. Perhaps they had a bitter disposition. Maybe they just didn't like you or had no interest in you. This is what somebody who does not smile communicates to the world around them. How happy can a person actually be if they can't smile? What sort of relationships can this person have without smiling, without communicating approval or happiness to the world? Indeed, this is the kind of person whom we often shun or try to stay away from.

If you could smile freely, what would you would be communicating to the world? How would your relationships be? Your relationship at the office, with your partner, when meeting people, with your friends, with strangers? And what would this do for your confidence? It is true that the first thing that people look at within the first five seconds of meeting you is your smile. What a better way of communication than a smile? Think about it. You don't even have to speak the same language. It is universal. Every single person on the planet including yourself should walk around with one of these, don't you think? This may take some getting used to if you've been afraid of the dentist for some time and you finally got a beautiful smile back, but a little adjustment time is worth showing the world your best side. And "best side" does mean your smile; there's a reason we say "million-dollar smile" and not "million-dollar earlobes."

How Much is this Going to Cost, Doc?

People avoid the dentist for a number of reasons, some of which have already been outlined: fear, lack of time, procrastination, and embarrassment are some common excuses. But there's another reason that people avoid the dentist altogether and that is financial. Whether you're afraid of the dentist or not, people want to spend the least amount of time as possible lying in a dental chair. I understand because I'm part of that group myself!

What I tell the person avoiding the dentist because of finances is this: no matter what your financial situation is, you're going to have to go to the dentist sooner or later. It is preferable to go sooner because basic dental treatment is exponentially less costly than major dental treatment. The cost of a basic white filling, for example, is a tenth of the cost of a root canal with a crown. The procedure takes one tenth of the time that it does to do a root canal and a crown, meaning that you're in a dental chair for a relatively short amount of time.

I also tell patients that the cost of procrastinating and avoiding the dentist is not only financial but also healthful. It is necessary that you keep your own natural teeth if at all possible. I can give you many examples, but for illustrative purposes the difference between dental implants and natural teeth is that with your own natural teeth you can feel what you have in between them when you are chewing, whereas with dental implants or dentures your ability to judge what you have been to your teeth and your chewing is virtually eliminated. Knowing that you are chewing something hard or soft and the awareness of knowing you need to continue chewing or the food in your mouth is ready to be swallowed makes chewing comfortable and efficient. Money may come and go, but sound health is invaluable and in many instances irreplaceable.

Some patients tell me that they want to wait until they get insurance to actually have their dental treatment done. The problem with dental insurance, though, is that it doesn't work like homeowner's insurance, automobile insurance or medical insurance. With all of these you pay a relatively small portion and the insurance company covers the rest. With dental insurance the opposite is true: they cover a very small percentage and you pay the rest. So if you want to take advantage of your dental insurance this year and wait until next year to complete another portion based on the fact that they cover small percentages,, By and large, though, it is not possible to make those ends meet and there will always be a deficit with respect to your oral health if you get it treated in fits and starts. When it comes to the financial aspects of acquiring sound oral health for life, it is better to pay the cost of treatment out of pocket than to wait years for insurance to pay for your dental treatment. Besides the frustration of living with dental problems for years while you wait for the money to come through, in most cases your potential problems can actually get worse in the meantime, requiring still more treatment (and money)!

In sum, let's just say that the cost of not going to the dentist can be somewhat more profound than getting and staying healthy. Keeping up with your oral health can help prevent weight gain, bad breath, and poor sleep (which might explain why most dentists are so devastatingly handsome). **More seriously, the cost of preventing or finding oral cancer or other dangerous conditions on time is worth your life.**

3

WHAT IS SEDATION DENTISTRY
AND DO I NEED IT?

*"I learned to be with myself rather than avoiding
myself with limiting habits; I started to be aware
of my feelings more, rather than numb them."*

— JUDITH WRIGHT

I opened my first dental practice the same year I graduated from dental school and I soon started to encounter something that I had not seen before, much less know how to handle it, even though I had attended one of the best dental schools in the world. You see, back when I started, the regular policy was for a general dentist to refer a patient who was terrified of the dentist to a specialist. That was the standard. Yes, some of us could administer laughing gas, but for a great deal of patients it just was not enough.

The problem with referring the patient was that it was a good way for dentists to get rid of patients who were uncomfortable to treat, but it presented a dilemma for both the patient and for me professionally. For the patient, this solution provided one of two options; remove the tooth or do nothing. The referred specialist was typically an oral surgeon who could not do a filling or fix a tooth. Their only option was to remove a "semi-problematic" tooth. Notice that this practice is not typically performed in other fields of medicine (when was the last time you heard about a surgeon who decided to pull out a "semi-problematic" brain?).

The problem with this for me was that as the person charged with the task of maintaining the patient's oral health sound for life, I could not afford to have a patient remove a generally healthy tooth. It was not only a detriment for the patient, but with fewer natural teeth, the task of maintaining a patient's oral health would become more cumbersome, less ideal, less comfortable and sub-optimal in general. This could present a lifelong problem for their general health as well.

Moreover, I found that a great deal of patients were pointing out something in my bedside manner that I found perplexing. In fact, to this day, it is still a mystery. It turns out that patients were making a big deal about **my** not making a big deal that they hadn't been to the dentist in quite a long time as a result of their fear. They were relieved and happy that I did not even mention it. What was commonplace and expected by the patient was to go to the dentist, finally confronting their fear, only to have the dentist lecture or berate them for their hand in their poor oral health!

Are you kidding me? How would that help at all? Plus, aren't we all afraid of something?! I don't blame anyone for being afraid of the dentist, heck frankly, I would be too if I wasn't one. Remember, you should be proud of going to the dentist, especially if you're dentophobic; under no circumstances should you feel ashamed to go to the dentist.

By 2001 I categorized several characteristics about the fearful patient. To my surprise, I've found that every fearful patient who's walked through my door was convinced that they had to be sedated to get through a dental appointment. Typical statements I've heard from fearful patients in my years of experience include:

> "I am your worst patient, Doc. You've never had a patient as bad as me!"
> "I need to be totally knocked out."
> "I can't get numb. My last dentist told me that he couldn't give me any more novocaine" (the solution to this later on in Chapter 4)
> "My last dentist told me that the pain I was feeling was all in my head" – I could agree with the dentist here inasmuch as the

mouth is on the part of the body commonly known as 'the head.'
"I had a dentist pull my teeth without novocaine."
"I'm terrified of needles."
"I am so embarrassed."

Some patients had indeed had bad experiences at the dentist that kept them from returning.

These were patients avoiding social interaction or covering their mouth when they laughed. Some men sported heavy mustaches. These patients tended to be heavy either from borderline depression or from tolerating only soft, high-caloric foods. In most cases, these patients were self-deprecating and ashamed.

Surprisingly, I discovered that my best patients, the ones who would forever comply with the necessary recommendations, the ones who would refer their friends and family and who were the most appreciative and happy, were the ones who had not been to the dentist in years because of fear. Patience and understanding, a lot of both, took my relationships with patients to great heights, but there was still the issue of the very high-fear ones. There was only so much I could do.

I decided that it was my responsibility to create the solution for people who avoid the dentist because of fear of the dentist, fear of pain and needles or bad past experiences. So with much criticism from peers, I invested considerable time in learning the science of sedation dentistry, and was vilified by colleagues when I made it available in my community. You see, dentists by and large are arguably very conservative, so when someone in their community starts to do something they themselves won't do, their feathers get ruffled. I still see this today. Perhaps it's human nature and perhaps it is the same in every profession. But, someone had to do something for these patients and I wasn't about to let "human nature" get in the way of providing the skills, expertise and tools necessary to get people who were terrified of the dentist to sound oral health.

Fast forward almost two decades later. Not only has sedation dentistry become mainstream in my community, not only have we apprenticed some of the most well-known sedation dentists in our community but over 35,000 patients have walked through our doors to avail themselves of anxiety-free dentistry. The end result of this effort is systems created for everyone to acquire and keep sound oral health, from the mildly apprehensive to the most terrified of patients to special needs patients.

So what is sedation dentistry? There are various forms of dental sedation. To clarify, dental anesthesia is what is used so that you don't feel any pain during the procedure, whereas the role of dental sedation involves allaying fear and apprehension with or without the use of drugs so that dentistry can be performed. Anesthesia and sedation are sometimes confused and interchanged by patients.

Let's examine a few of the forms of sedation that might be used in dentistry:

Iatrosedation

My preferred form of sedation and inherently necessary for success in nearly every doctor-patient relationship is a technique known as iatrosedation. The etymology of the word "Iatro" is the Greek word "iatros" meaning physician. It means "related to a physician" and used as a prefix means "induced or caused by a physician." Iatrosedation, a term I first learned from world-renowned sedation dentist and academic Dr. Stanley Malamed at the beginning of my career, means to sedate a patient simply by way of communication and without pharmaceuticals. It is not hypnosis or anything of the sort. It is interview-based and takes a fearful or apprehensive patient to a point where he or she is no longer controlled by their dental-related fears to the point where he or she can cope with the experience.

By and large, the vast majority of patients who once had to be sedated with medications when their treatment began no longer require it as a result of iatrosedation; although drug-induced sedation allows the trained dentist to complete much-needed treatment in few visits, well-implemented iatrosedation allows the fearful patient to actually "cure," or at least begin to handle, their overwhelming fear so that pharmacosedation is not necessary in subsequent and maintenance visits.

There are various methods of inducing sedation in high fear dental patients with medications and in the interest of your understanding I will cut through the medical jargon. There are various forms of drug induced dental sedation and here they are broken up into two simple categories: those administered directly into the blood stream and those that are administered through other methods.

"Laughing Gas"

One of the simplest forms of allaying dental fears is by way of nitrous oxide, commonly known as laughing gas. Although nitrous oxide gas is considered an anesthetic, that is, a pain-eliminating agent, it is a very weak anesthetizing agent when administered by the methods in which it is used today, and it is an ideal sedative for the mildly to moderately anxious patient. In yesteryear, this agent was used without the use of oxygen. When the patient began to turn cyanotic and blue, the physician would go to work. This of course was not the safest of uses, and like most gas sedative agents it allowed the operator a very narrow window for performing a procedure. Nowadays, the use of nitrous oxide gas is concomitantly administered with oxygen, and most nitrous oxide machines are used with a governor, a fixed mechanism that does not allow the nitrous oxide gas to exceed 70% of the gas being inhaled, the rest of the mixture of course being oxygen. It gets a person feeling relaxed, some like if they had a couple of beers, others like if they had three six-packs. The goal is to get the patient sufficiently relaxed to a fine point and balance described later. By the way, you will hear me repeat over and over again in this section that it is necessary to discuss the risks, options, benefits and alternatives for sedation and your particular circumstances with your dentist, but I can assure you right now that if you are afraid of embarrassing yourself with laughing uncontrollably in front of complete strangers, don't worry! Such situations are not likely to happen in any event. I would estimate that of two hundred patients who are administered laughing gas, maybe two experience laughing fits, and if they do it lasts 30-60 seconds at most.

Like any form of sedation or anxiety-allaying agent, under the right hands nitrous oxide is a relatively safe method of handling fear and anxiety. It goes without saying that whatever the method of sedation, drug-induced anxiety reducer or anesthetic, a thorough explanation (not included in this book) should be sought from your dentist prior to its use so that you are accurately informed of the risks associated with any drug before you consent to its use. It is up to your dentist and you to decide on what form of sedation is most practical for you after a thorough discussion of the risks, benefits and alternatives available for you which are beyond the scope of this book.

It's As Easy As Taking A Pill

All right, that chapter heading is meant to be tongue-in-cheek. I am not in favor of using medication where it can be avoided. When it is necessary, though, the next form of sedation, a step above nitrous oxide gas, is the use of sedatives in the form of pills. A vast array of pill and tablet medications are available that will allow the dentist to work for two to five hours while you are relaxed, or even completely dozed off. There are pros and cons to pill sedation, but the central drawback is that a swallowed pill or tablet, unlike intravenous sedation where the medication is delivered directly into the blood, while being transported from the gastrointestinal system into the blood stream, has to pass through the liver where its effect starts to diminish. It is thus not as easy for the clinician to evaluate exactly how large of a dose to administer in pill or tablet form to give to achieve the desired effect.

There are other risks that the dentist will let you know about prior to using pills or any other form of sedation. Some of the benefits of pill sedation are that it is ideal for patients who are absolutely terrified of needles. This makes it more tolerable to some. Pill form sedation can also be used in conjunction with nitrous oxide gas to better control the state of sedation and find that sweet spot that will have the patient comfortably sedated while having their teeth rehabilitated. One of the benefits that patients appreciate is that, depending on the medication used, there is typically little to no recollection of the procedure and the patient feels like they slept through the entire procedure. Of course, catching up on your beauty sleep in the chair also means missing out on the chance to really address the fear that kept you out of that chair in the first place.

Intravenous Sedation

Taking the level of sedation up a couple of notches is intravenous sedation. As mentioned earlier and as the name suggests, these drugs are administered directly into the bloodstream to achieve a level of sedation and anxiety reduction. As already mentioned, there are risks associated with this and any form of sedation, and that goes double for forms that are delivered directly into the bloodstream as their effects can be profound and immediate. While more powerful, IV sedation can also be safer for patients to achieve a more immediate sedation. This is because the dentist has a better method for regulating based on clinical judgement how much more medication to give depending on the required treatment and desired sedative effect. Administered correctly, IV sedation allows patients to feel like they slept through their treatment.

It should be noted, although it seems obvious, that the more profound the effect of a medication used, the less safe it can be or the more complicated the operation can be. This is why I really prefer iatrosedation, because the patient is much more comfortable than prior to their dental experience. While iatrosedation can act as a cure for fear of the dentist, pharmacosedation is more of a band-aid for their fear so that they can get through their visit without actually addressing the root cause of their fear.

I want to make a very important point here.

Ninety percent of patients that come to me because they are afraid of the dentist tell me that they want to be "out" during their treatment and that they just want to wake up when everything is over, awaking to healthy teeth.

While this is understandable and the ideal scenario in an ideal world, the fact is that by and large, the less sedated a person is the more comfortable they may really be. The more sedated a person is, the more cumbersome it is to perform dental treatment on them. It's a fine line to walk, and a sweet spot must be found. This sweet spot is the goal of sedation dentistry for the clinician: achieving that target where the patient is comfortable because their fear has been controlled and performing their dental treatment in a way that is comfortable for them. Moreover, the less medication used, the safer it may be for the patient. I use a word "may" because every situation is different, and for example a patient with high blood pressure may benefit from more sedative agents in order to maintain their blood pressure control during the procedure. But the general fact remains that the less medication that can be practically administered, the safer it is for the patient. Remember that arguably the most critical risk with sedation is maintaining an open airway so the patient can breathe normally and maintain their blood oxygen saturation at a normal level. This is one of the many things that must be discussed with your doctor prior to any sedation.

Deep Sedation

Having said this there is another, still more profound form of sedation: general anesthesia. General anesthesia has its uses in sedation dentistry and it is mainly for use in the most difficult cases. Of course, "difficult" is a relative term. What may be difficult for another dentist may not be difficult for me. This is evidence by the fact that I treat special needs patients – that is, patients with Down syndrome, autism, cerebral palsy, or Alzheimers – and the use of general anesthesia is the exception even with these patients. I treat these patients in the office with or without conscious sedation, the type of sedation described previously where the patient becomes alert with a simple stimulus on my part. This is something to keep in mind the next time you feel that visiting the dentist is impossible!

There is a place, however, for general anesthesia. While I can treat 99.9% of high-fear patients with conscious sedation, a very small percentage, including special needs patients or medically compromised patients, do require deep sedation or even general anesthesia. It should be noted that deep sedation is a form of sedation that lies between conscious sedation and general anesthesia and requires special permitting by most state regulatory agencies, as do conscious sedation and general anesthesia. Deep sedation and general anesthesia can be performed in an outpatient facility, although certain situations may call for a hospital setting.

I have simplified the various forms of sedation in this section for the sake of a general explanation, but it is necessary to discuss the risks, benefits and alternatives in your particular case with your doctor as they have not all been fully described here. You should also note that I have not alluded to any safety regarding sedation, anesthesia or dental treatment. While the need for safety is obvious to you the educated reader, we live in a society where we have to resort to disclaimers for things that are obvious, even in a car commercial where a car is flying out the window of a skyscraper into the next building – "Closed course and professional driver... Don't try this at home..." You get the point. Sedation in any situation, or even the use of appropriately used medications, can be dangerous. Get the lowdown from your doctor before doing anything.

4

HOW CAN I GET MY TEETH FIXED WITHOUT PAIN?

"Courage is resistance to fear, mastery of fear – not absence of fear. Except a creature be part coward it is not compliment to say it is brave."

— MARK TWAIN

Up until now I've discussed several ways in which a person who is mildly afraid or terrified can be helped through a dental procedure. As previously discussed however sedation and not feeling pain are two totally different things. Remember, sedation is used to allay fear and apprehension while anesthesia is used to eliminate the possibility of feeling pain. Having thoroughly examined the former, let's take a closer look at anesthesia.

Since the time of the ancient Egyptians, a battle has been fought for healing teeth without pain. Yet almost

4000 years later, people are still avoiding dental care because they are afraid of the possible pain they may feel at the dentist. I would like to point out that the primary medical procedure performed back then involved drilling a hole in the patient's skull to let out the evil spirits, so I'd like to think we've at least made a *little* progress.

If you hate the dental drill or if you hate having your teeth picked on with metal tools, I have some great news for you in upcoming chapters. But first, let's look at how to get your teeth fixed without pain.

I can't tell you how often a patient comes to me saying "novocaine does not work on me and I have a hard time getting numb."

This then is followed by "I once had a dentist do a root canal [or filling] and I felt everything. The dentist gave me ten shots and finally told me that he couldn't give me any more, that it was impossible that I was feeling any pain, that it was all in my head."

I follow this up by asking the patient if the tooth that was being treated at the time was a lower back tooth and ten out of ten times the answer is "yes." You see, by my own account 85% of patients who are having a lower back tooth treated will indeed successfully get numb with the standard technique of anesthetizing taught in dental school, which leaves a relatively large 15% of patients having their tooth treated without functional anesthetic. It is no doubt why patient after patient complains that he felt pain with his last dentist which in turn kept him from going to the dentist again. It is because the vast majority of dentists only know how to anesthetize with the standard technique they learned in dental school, a technique that by my own observation does not work and is ineffective in 15% to 20% of the public as a result of variations in the position of the nerve that needs to be blocked with anesthesia.

Although I've tried to give as little technical information in this text as possible, I'm going to give you some additional information that I'm going to show you how to use later on in the book so that when you go to the dentist can be assured that you won't encounter any pain. A small caveat is necessary here: remember the mixed martial arts behemoth that I told you about earlier on in the book? There is a perception component to pain as well as the physical aspect, and that is not treated by anesthetic. However, using the information that you will have in your arsenal by the end of this book, you will be able to handle the component of perception as well.

If you don't want to have or go through pain when having your lower jaw teeth treated, there are two techniques that your dentist can use. One is called the Gow-Gates Block and the other is called the Akinazi-Vazirani Block. The former was touted and mystified by oral surgeon instructors in dental school as a technique exclusive to oral surgeons but that had to be learned in theory by all dentists. The second technique I had not even heard of until after I graduated. Both are effective techniques that successfully anesthetize patients 99.9% of the time. I use them almost exclusively as they are not only more effective than the standard block, but they actually bother every patient less during administering. Using these techniques makes it almost impossible to feel pain while having a dental procedure done. Yes, really!

And what if you're in that fraction of a percent who still can't get numb because of an extraordinary variant in the way your nerves are positioned? Don't worry, we still have you covered. There is a virtually painless system of delivering the anesthetic directly in the area where the tooth is that will get it numb. It's called "The X-Tip." If this too doesn't work then you may be a candidate for deep or general anesthesia, but in almost twenty years of practice I have never encountered this problem.

That's Really Enlightening, Doc...but I'm Afraid of Needles!

This is where sedation comes in: to get you to a point where you don't realize what's going on. But as I have repeatedly mentioned, I like to try everything in my arsenal before resorting to drugs.

What if I told you, perception of pain aside, that you could be numbed without pain?

One of the systems that I have created addresses specifically the distaste that comes with getting a shot. The first thing that needs to be addressed is, of course, a patient's fear of needles. You will learn my system for handling this by the end of the book, but because I have so many ways of addressing fear I always like to ask the patient, "Do you know what caused you to fear needles?"

Sometimes the patient tells me they were injected many times during a futile effort on the part of the dentist to get him or her numb. Others tell me that it hurts them terribly. Still others can't tell me why they are afraid of needles, and that's ok. It's a common response. Needles hurt! You no more need to explain why you're afraid of them than you need to explain why you're not a fan of falling from great heights.

The second thing that my system addresses is the actual pinch of the needle. I can tell you that for us men this is the worst part, no matter how big, brave, and valiant we are (or claim to be). My system handles this in three parts. First, a special type of cream anesthetic is used to numb the skin. I was never a proponent of this topical anesthetic because I found it to be useless in the past and served more of a psychological comforter, until I discovered an effective formula of ingredients within the cream that does indeed provide a profound and noticeable anesthesia.

But that's not all. I don't like to run the risk of possible pain when I'm anesthetizing so after the topical anesthetic has taken effect, I use an instrument that overrides pain receptors in the area that will be anesthetized by use of vibration. It looks like an electric toothbrush and when I place it on the area where the injection will occur, it subtly vibrates, it tickles a bit, but it keeps the pinch from hurting, and by most accounts the injection is not even felt.

The usefulness of this instrument in keeping a patient from feeling injections is truly remarkable and is one of my favorite tools in my pain-free injection arsenal. The third component of the painless anesthesia system so the pinch is not felt is the use of special needles (sorry, I just had to use the word). These are extraordinarily small in diameter and minimize any discomfort even in the absence of the other components.

Now that the pinch has been addressed, the delivery of the anesthesia may still be uncomfortable, even painful. There are various reasons for this and one of them is the temperature of the anesthesia. Room temperature is normally 75 degrees Fahrenheit while body temperature is 98.6. This difference in temperature can be very uncomfortable, so in my practice we warm the anesthetic to minimize discomfort. But what causes the most discomfort or pain when being anesthetized is the pH of the anesthetic itself. You see, some of the more effective anesthetics have a component in it that makes it difficult for the anesthesia to wear out. This is beneficial so that you don't have to be injected over and over again and allows for longer procedures to be performed. It's better to be numbed once and have many fillings performed at once for example than to complete them piecemeal or being injected routinely and more often. Fewer shots are generally better than more, I'm sure you'll agree!

But this ingredient of the anesthetic that makes its effect last longer requires a preservative, and this preservative is acidic. This is one of the greatest causes of pain when being anesthetized. This is easily overcome first by using an anesthetic that doesn't contain this component, then by following it up with the regular anesthesia once the area is numb, and by buffering or neutralizing the acid just before giving the injection. While pain is relative (indeed worse for the guys than the gals -they are stronger and I'm not just trying to win brownie points here), the system, composed of possible gas or other sedation if necessary, the special block technique, the topical anesthetic, the small needle, the vibrating instrument, the regulation of the temperature of the anesthetic, and the acid buffer brings peace of mind to my high-fear patients, setting the mood for the rest of the dental procedure.

I personally dislike the feeling of being numb or the feeling of pins and needles when it is wearing off, so I also offer my patients a reversal agent for the anesthetic. Although it doesn't reverse the anesthesia instantly, instead of three to six hours the numbness starts to disappear in thirty minutes, making the patient comfortable and ready for whatever else they need to do throughout the day (eating, for example, is a personal favorite of mine).

5

WHAT OTHER DENTAL TOOLS ARE AVAILABLE TO MAKE MY DENTAL EXPERIENCE COMFORTABLE?

"Technology is nothing. What's important is that you have a faith in people, that they're basically good and smart, and if you give them tools, they'll do wonderful things with them."

— STEVE JOBS

Once upon a time, the idea of making dental treatment comfortable was an oxymoron. You've discovered the various innovations and system that make painful novocaine injections in dentistry a thing of the past. Now let's get into the fancy gadgets available to make your experience more relaxing and more comfortable.

You Know the Drill

Who likes the sound of the drill? I'm not a fan of it, either, and...well, I'm a dentist! For one, it's annoying as heck working all day listening to that. But I'm not the one with the whining drill by my face, it's you. Since removing dental decay becomes efficient with a drill as opposed to scooping it up with a special instrument that then leaves decay behind and takes forever and a day to complete, the drill is a necessary evil in dentistry. There is, however, an alternative to the high-pitched sound that sends shivers up the spine of patients: it's called the electric handpiece.

The electric handpiece, as the name suggests, runs on electricity and not compressed air. It thus has several benefits. First, it is quiet. When your dentist uses an electric handpiece, you won't have a whining, high-pitched tool next to your face. Secondly, like an electric car which doesn't have a lag when pressing the accelerator, the efficiency of the electric handpiece is furthered by the fact that its spin or rotation does not diminish when it comes in contact with your tooth. What this means to you is that not only is it quiet but the procedure is completed quicker than with the older regular drills. Less time in the dental chair is always preferable, right?

Another alternative to drills is the use of a sandblasting instrument. This instrument removes decay by sandblasting the affected parts of the tooth. Some of the benefits of this instrument are less noise than a drill and less probability of heating the tooth, thus reduced pain should the patient not be correctly anesthetized. The drawback of this instrument, however, is that it normally takes longer to remove decay than with a handpiece and thus increases your time in the dental chair.

How Can Lasers In Dentistry Impact Comfort at the Dentist and Fear of Pain?

"As fun as picking at your teeth with a sharp metal instrument" is not something that anyone has ever said. Again, I personally dislike metal touching my teeth. Enter the cavity-detecting laser. Put simply, this is a laser that can detect cavities by way of light instead of the dentist having to pick at your teeth. What's even better is that the laser light bouncing off the tooth tells the doctor how deep or shallow the cavity is by way of a sound. Although there may be an exception to everything, this procedure is also completely painless.

While doing some research in 2004, I came across a video of a laser whose designers touted could reverse the bone loss associated with gum disease...at least, that was my understanding of it at the time. It has always been a medical fact that bone loss around teeth, periodontitis or gum disease described earlier in Chapter 2, is irreversible. I immediately thought, "If these claims are true, it will revolutionize dentistry!" Well, I am proud to report that in 2004, I embraced and introduced in my county the only FDA-approved laser alternative to gum surgery. With this alternative there's no need for scalpels, no need for cutting, no need for stitches and rarely any pain or discomfort following the procedure. Compared to the decades-held standard for addressing severe bone loss around teeth, which was a particular technique that's... well, a bit graphic to describe. The choice seems pretty obvious, right? What's more, with the laser technique we can regain some of the lost bone back. The procedure which has achieved tremendous success for countless of patients who suffered from periodontal disease is called LANAP and its benefits over other alternatives are exponential.

Other Tools and Gadgets

There's an LED-based instrument (which is not a laser) used in combating cancer that is worth mentioning. I have come across oral cancer both in patients who regularly frequent the dentist as well as those who don't. This instrument looks like a flashlight and is called a **Velscope**. The Velscope helps the dentist with the visualization of infections, cancer, pre-cancer, tumors and other illnesses. As should be obvious by now, I am a firm believer that not going to the dentist can hurt you in many ways, and this instrument makes it easier for you to remain healthy. There's not one oral examination I do that doesn't include an oral cancer screening.

Digital x-rays in dentistry have been around for well over 25 years and have been fine-tuned ever since. Digital x-rays present various benefits over traditional cardboard x-rays. For one thing, biting on a cardboard x-ray film can be painful. Moreover, traditionally if an x-ray is taken and found to be inadequate after waiting fifteen minutes for development, another film had to be taken, which can be irritating for patient and dentist alike. What should be a simple process took the clinician and patient thirty minutes without the procedure even starting, and that was just one film!

Digital x-rays are more comfortable to hold in the mouth than cardboard film, develop in five seconds instead of fifteen minutes, and reduce radiation exposure by 90%. What does this mean to you? Other than the obvious benefits, it reduces root canal and treatment time significantly; as a result of this and other gadgets, most root canals now take an hour or so to complete as opposed to two or three visits. This is significant in many respects including increased comfort, cost reduction and health-related benefits. Moreover, digital x-rays minimize the effect of regular film x-rays which contain lead and require harmful environmental chemicals for developing. And hey, if digital film is good enough for your Facebook profile, surely it's good enough for your mouth!

I am certain that by now you may have become a bit less timid about finally getting to the dentist. I will soon give you a surefire method for incorporating what you have learned so far and what is to come so that you can comfortably have your dental treatment starting with the very first visit.

6

IF ONLY I COULD JUST GET PAST THE EMBARRASSMENT OF NEGLECTING MYSELF AND THE CONDITION OF MY TEETH

"We're often afraid of looking at our shadow because we want to avoid the shame or embarrassment that comes along with admitting mistakes."

— MARIANNE WILLIAMSON

This topic is so important and the problem so rampant that I have dedicated an entire chapter to addressing it. I take the liberty of doing so because it is a primary motivator that keeps people who have avoided the dentist away. Embarrassment is a natural human emotion common to all of us, much the same way fear is. It is a self-conscious distress that is effected when we are aware that others are aware or may become aware of our mistakes or slip-ups or when we anticipate that we may slip up before others. To some degree, embarrassment keeps us from making the same mistakes over and over again, and in one way or another it communicates to others that we are aware of and recognize our blunder or error.

More often than not shame, a similar emotion, may be related to avoiding the dentist. People whose health may have deteriorated as a result of avoiding the dentist are aware of their error. The emotion that typically follows is shame. Unlike embarrassment, the error of our ways is at hand but not shared with others and is living within us. Our errors can also lead us to guilt, where the focus is solely on what error we've made. These are all reasons people who have avoided the dentist propagate the situation. It is a vicious circle that, as previously discussed, affects one's health, self-esteem, relationships, work, happiness, and life in general and not for the better!

In avoiding the dentist the first behavior that usually comes is the direct or indirect fear-causing occurrence, then there is unsurmountable fear, avoidance of the dentist, deterioration of health, an awareness of not having gone to the dentist, increased avoidance, an even greater fear, ever-increased deterioration and so on and so on. It is a cycle that worsens and worsens, and as I've previously mentioned, one will inevitably confront the dentist sooner or later. Better sooner.

Justification is a mechanism we use to make right even our biggest wrongs right. No one likes to think of themselves as anything less than right and good. The husband who cheats on his wife has to make his error okay to himself, otherwise guilt, the focus on his error, may set in. He justifies it, tries to ameliorate his transgression, by blaming her for not cooking, her lack of intimacy or her ranting about not leaving his socks next to the bed. The child who steals a pencil justifies his transgression ok, justifies, by telling the teacher Billy did it first and thus Billy made him do it. While it is easy to sing our own praises, it takes quite a bit of conscientiousness and know-how to really look at our actions and accept oneself as the cause of a sub-optimal effect or error.

I am not suggesting that avoiding the dentist because of embarrassment or fear is a great gaffe, but it is a form of transgression against oneself. The conscious awareness that we are doing something that may be harmful to us is in itself a self-transgression and we do tend to justify these as well. I hear patients on occasion say that they need to discuss things with their spouse, yet they haven't been to the dentist in decades. Patients tell me they don't have time or can't afford treatment, yet they spend on their children's cell phone bills, cable TV, and a vacation. There are many ways one justifies and makes right their continued neglect of their health. It is the easier thing to do.

Now, I understand it from the patient's perspective, but now it's time for you to understand it from mine. There's not a week that goes by when I'm not embarrassed about something myself. There's not a month that goes by when I don't have my attention on a blunder of my own, and indeed I too focus in on some of those mistakes that I've made throughout my life. I have done some great things in my life but I have screwed up royally as well. You and I and everyone has. If you can name me one sentient adult who has not made one error in his life then please let me know. Life cannot occur without error. This is how we learn, this is how we grow, and this is how we keep from repeating an error. The perfection that is life lies in that it is imperfect.

The dentist who made you feel wrong, who lectured you to the end of embarrassing you and making you more aware that he/she was aware of your error, thereby in-validating you...this dentist did you no favor, and in fact did you a real disservice.

Invalidation is the act of making one smaller. I am of the most firm conviction that pointing out a patient's error does nothing but introvert a patient, especially when done in an emotionally charged environment like that of a dental operatory,. Getting the patient to look in (that is, introvert) at the error sitting there in the top of his mind? That causes nothing but embarrassment. How does this empower a person the dentist supposedly cares for? By the same token, I am of the most firm conviction that a person who has avoided the dentist because of fear must be validated. It take nerve and guts to confront fear and embarrassment, and I don't know about you but I am not immune to any of these. I admire guts. I know my end and that of the patient's in this doctor-patient relationship.

If you are ready to confront your fear count on me to be your leader and we will get through it together, tete-a-tete, shoulder to shoulder. Let me introduce you to the Piedra Method so you can start to make real, immediate progress towards conquering your fear of the dentist.

7

THE PIEDRA METHOD: 5 EASY STEPS TOWARD HEALTHY TEETH AND GUMS FOR A LIFETIME FOR THE HIGH-FEAR PATIENT

"Every great and deep difficulty bears in itself its own solution. It forces us to change our thinking in order to find it."

— NIELS BOHR

The goal of any sedation dentist should be to get the patient to sound oral health and maintenance for life, comfortably and without the use of sedation or sedatives. In dentistry, it is necessary to actively have the participation of the patient. For us to work together successfully we need voluntary movement of the head in different positions: voluntary opening, voluntary closing, and so on. Not sedating a patient makes the procedure shorter and more efficient for both opera-tor and patient. Sedation takes time to take effect and voluntary cooperation of the patient is limited, making the procedure longer (as discussed in Chapter 3). A fine balance of comfort and practicality for the patient can to be achieved.

The Piedra Method

Step One: Getting Past the Front Door

Call the dentist before driving to the first consultation. If you are very afraid or em-barrassed of going to the dentist, call up the dental office and arrange to speak on the phone with the dentist. The difficulty gradient is greatly diminished by doing this over when going in for an initial consulta-tion. Explain to the dentist that you haven't been in for years, that you had a bad experi-ence. As discussed, shame and embarrass-ment are common reasons for high-fear patients to avoid going, so this is a good time to let the dentist know how you feel. Believe me, we don't distinguish one bad tooth from fifteen bad teeth! At this point, make certain to make it clear to the dentist that you are aware of the need to go rou-tinely, that you're finally getting in despite your fear, and that you absolutely do not want to be lectured.

Step Two: Getting Past the Injection

A purported 78% of the public is afraid of needles...and understandably so! Many report that they had experiences at a dentist where the dentist gave them ten shots and they were still not numb. Refer to chapter 4 for a thorough explanation on how to overcome this.

The reason this person could not get numb is because 15-20% of the public, when being anesthetized for a bottom back tooth, cannot get numb with the conventional method of numbing these teeth that are taught in dental school, known as an Inferior Alveolar Nerve Block. This will work on 80-85% of patients

During Step One, in your initial telephone dialogue with the dentist, ask how he or she addresses the subject of needles, fear of needles, and fear of pain. If he doesn't tell you outright that he buffers the anesthetic, that he uses the thinnest needle available, that he uses a vibrating instrument and if you still feel comfortable with the dialogue that you've had so far, ask him if he is willing to provide all of the above. These things should be commonplace in every dental practice but indeed are unfortunately the exception.

By the way, it merits reiterating that some patients afraid of needles may be equally or relatively afraid or uncomfortable with that picking instrument we call the "explorer." Indeed, I am one of those who really dislikes having a pointy, metallic tool scraping my tooth while being checked for cavities. If this sounds like you, recall the laser from Chapter 5 and ask the dentist if he uses a cavity-detecting laser. Again, diagnostic lasers in the examination process can detect cavities, the size and depth of the cavity, and are completely painless; a godsend to many patients and for the dentist as well!

Step Three: I am in Control Here

Unlike Alexander Haig, at the dentist it is quite all right to assume control. One of the most difficult things for most people to do, let alone people afraid of the dentist, is to remain calm while lying face-up in a supine and vulnerable position while a stranger works in close proximity to the part of the body where you breathe, the part that allows you to see and hear. The sound of the whining drill, the smell of cloves and eugenol, the bright light in your face, the tactical feeling of another person's hand in your mouth...All senses are stimulated while a complete stranger works on you with intimidating, high pitched sounds and sharp tools...This is unnerving for anyone!

The problem generally lies in the feeling that the dentist and his tools are completely in control and one is completely helpless. This is a very bad feeling of not being in control and at the mercy of someone else.

For this reason, I always tell the patient to lift their left hand should they need me to stop for WHATEVER reason. Whether there's too much water for their comfort, whether they feel something is uncomfortable, whether they anticipate something and want to bring it to my attention....whatever it is, I tell the patient to lift their left hand and stop me as many times as necessary and to not worry about how many times I am stopped.

Extraordinary yet simple communication is what is necessary here, and believe me, this will make things easier for the dentist himself, too, so don't be shy to communicate. During your initial consultation, come to an agreement with your dentist. Be straightforward and tell him that this is difficult and that you would like to be able to communicate freely with him during the procedure and ask if it is okay with him if you lift your hand in order to stop him and communicate with him. Believe me, this is much better and more productive for him than to have you rigid in fear or expectation and moaning. This will make your job and his job easier. Believe me, you will be much more at ease knowing you can stop at will and take a breather if you need to.

Step Four: The Referral

I have found that after four dental visits, high-fear patients normally starts to feel significantly much more comfortable. Remember Iatrosedation? The goal is for you, the patient, not to be afraid, not to require any sedation to be able to have your dental treatment performed. Patients who complete this Method normally become advocates of fearlessness at the dentist and become excellent sources of referrals. I would ask the dentist of names and phone numbers of patients who have had similar experiences as yours but were able to get through dental procedure. You would be surprised as to how many people are actually afraid to one degree or the another of the dentist and were able to surpass their fear. The insight that these healthy patients can offer is much more than any dentist or any book can offer, as I have found that patients benefit tremendously from speaking with others who have gone through what they're going through...

Step Five: The Parachute (Be Prepared)

Be prepared is not only the Boy Scout motto, but something to keep in mind before going to the dentist...and I don't mean to be prepared to bail out! What I do mean is that you should be prepared in case you do start to have overwhelming feeling of fear during a dental procedure. The first action to take, of course, is to lift your left hand and stop the procedure. The next step is to recognize that something unknown from the past has been re-stimulated and

is causing you to have a fight-or-flight re-
flex activate.

Next, the key thing to do is to immediately start to look at details in your surroundings and notice things that you have not noticed before. Look at one thing you have not noticed before. Feel something you haven't felt before, like for example, the feeling of your back on the chair. Then look at something far away and notice something about it that you haven't noticed before. Then move on to something close. What do you smell that you haven't smelled before? What do you hear that you had not noticed? All of these things, done enough, will get your fight-or-flight to deactivate, removing the unconscious culprit that is making you react to a conscious aware-ness you're in a different place and time as though you are in the dangerous situation that your body and mind learned to react from. Do this until you are comfortable. This actually works in most situations where the emotion you're having is not the one the moment calls for, such as when you suddenly are fearful, anxious, or worried without real cause.

By making use of the Piedra Method you will accomplish two key elements in living a life of healthy teeth and gums. Now that you know what is at your disposal so that you don't ever relive the whining sound of a dental drill, pain-ful injections and painful procedures or embarrassment you have at your reach the wherewithal to personally surpass that which kept you from sound oral health and a tool to put you in a position of *cause* with regard to the dentist as opposed to one of *effect*.

Conclusion

> *"The opposite of bravery is not cowardice but conformity."*

> — ROBERT ANTHONY

We've talked about many different ways in which modern dentistry and specialized systems can transform your fear of dentists, needles, pain or embarrassment and make your dental experience tolerable and fearless. What's most critical to take away from this book is the Piedra Method, the method you have gained to get through the dentist and dental treatment fearlessly and comfortably.

Now I will leave you with the number-one secret to transforming your fear to bravery when it comes to the dentist, almost overnight:

It is only by pursuing a system that you can free yourself from further pain, oral and general disease, chaos, embarrassment, and even an inability to smile freely. Keeping in mind which instrumentation and dental bedside manner systems are available to you so that you don't have to go through painful dental procedures, painful injections or even embarrassing lectures, find a dentist who provides these techniques and systems to his or her patients. From here it all boils down now to taking the second step, your part of the process in transforming dental fear to bravery and gaining the sound oral health, aesthetics, confidence, and freedom you deserve: the Piedra Method.

If you would like a personal consultation with Dr. Rene Piedra, call 305-667-6747.